The cure for aging how to live long, young and healthy: Secrets to successful aging.

Dr Kc Thompson (PhD).

Table of contents

Chapter 1

What is aging?

Aging is a gradual, continuous process of natural change that begins in early adulthood. During early middle age, many bodily functions begin to gradually decline.

People do not become old or elderly at any specific age. Traditionally, age 65 has been designated as the beginning of old age. But the reason was based in history, not biology. Many years ago, age 65 was chosen as the age for retirement in Germany, the first nation to establish a retirement program. In 1965 in the United States, age 65 was designated as the eligibility age for Medicare insurance. This age is close to the actual retirement age of most people in economically advanced societies.

The 3 Unique Kinds of Aging.

Biological Aging.

This is the type of aging most people are familiar with, since it refers to the various ways the human body naturally changes over time. For instance, immune system changes associated with age make it more difficult to fight infections and viruses.

Biological aging can also affect digestion, the spine, joints, vital organs, and other parts that help with movement and daily functioning. Hearing, vision, and oral health can also be affected by biological issues. Biological aging is something that happens to everyone. However, seniors may be able to age well biologically by:

• Staying within a healthy weight range.
• Getting regular exercise.
 • Being proactive about recommended health screenings.
• Eating fresh fruits and veggies and other foods good for an aging body Seniors can face a variety of age-related challenges.

Though some families choose to take on the caregiving duties, there may come a time when they need a trusted home care provider. Families sometimes need respite from their duties so they can focus on their other responsibilities, and some seniors need around-the-clock assistance that their families are not able to provide. Home Care Assistance is here to help.

Psychological Aging.

This type of aging is largely related to behavior, but it also includes general perception and reactions to the immediate environment. Psychological aging is related to changes in the brain and, in some cases, underlying psychological issues or changes in cognitive capabilities that could affect problem-solving, emotions, and subjective reactions to situations. While there are many factors that could affect psychological aging, seniors tend to be better prepared to handle this aspect of aging with efforts that involve:

• Having healthy emotional outlets (e.g., friends/family members to talk to).
• Getting the support needed to manage unexpected life changes.
• Eating healthy foods that keep the brain mentally sharp.
• Treating signs of depression and similar disorders early Biological aspects of aging could also affect how an older adult ages psychologically.

For instance, if there are untreated issues with hearing or vision, an older adult's perception of the world may influence his or her behavior. Maintaining a high quality of life can be challenging for some seniors, but professional caregivers can help them obtain this goal. Families can trust a renowned homecare service experts to help their elderly loved ones focus on lifestyle choices that increase the chances of living a longer and healthier life.

Social Aging.

Social aging refers to how social habits and behaviors change over time. It also includes the individual's role in relation to society as a whole and people in his or her age group. This type of aging is measured, in part, by how an individual is expected to behave in interactions with others based on social norms. From available opportunities for social engagement to psychological issues and age-related cognitive changes, there are many factors that can influence social aging. That being said, there are some things seniors can do to age well socially.

Recommendations typically involve:

• Maintaining healthy relationships with friends and family members.
• Exploring new ways to socially engage as life circumstances change.
• Getting any assistance that may be needed to address physical limitations that could be affecting social interactions Aging in place can present a few unique challenges for older adults. Some only require part-time assistance with exercise or meal preparation, while others are living with serious illnesses and benefit more significantly from receiving live-in care. .

Chapter 2

Symptoms of aging

We all know the obvious signs of aging: wrinkles, gray hair, a slightly stooped posture, perhaps some "senior moments" of forgetfulness. But why do those things happen? What is aging?

Each of us is made up of cells—13 trillion of them. Our tissues and organs are each a bunch of cells, held together with various natural materials that the cells have made.

From the moment of conception, each of our cells—and, hence, our tissues and organs—begins a process of aging. Early in life, of course, we still are growing, and expanding the number of cells that we have. The cells are aging, but so slightly that we can't see it: we just see the body growing and developing.

At some point in life, often in the 30's, the tell-tale signs of aging begin to be apparent. They can be seen in everything from our vital signs (like blood pressure) to our skin, to our bone and joints, to our cardiovascular, digestive, and nervous systems, and beyond. Some aging changes begin early in life. For example, your metabolism starts to gradually decline beginning at about age 20. Changes in your hearing, on the other hand, do not usually begin until age 50 or later.

We do not yet fully understand the complex interplay of factors that cause us to age as we do. We know that many different things affect aging: genetics, diet, exercise, illness, and a host of other factors, all of which contribute to the aging process.

A series of remarkable biological research studies since the 1990's have identified genes that can profoundly influence the rate at which cells, and animals, age. The good news from these studies is that biological changes that extend life also seem to extend vitality: animals that live longer remain quite healthy for most of their lengthened life.

None of these discoveries is close to providing a "fountain of youth" for humans, but some scientists believe that research breakthroughs regarding aging in the 21st Century will lead to the development of drugs that can extend human life and simultaneously improve human health. If that happens, of course, it will only be a good thing if the world finds room, work and resources for all the additional people.

Symptoms:

We each age at different rates, and to different degrees, and yet we experience many common effects of aging. Some common signs and symptoms of aging include:

Increased susceptibility to infection

Greater risk of heat stroke or hypothermia

Slight decrease in height as the bones of our spines get thinner and lose some height

Bones break more easily

Joint changes, ranging from minor stiffness to severe arthritis

Stooped posture

Slowed and limited movement

Decrease in overall energy

Constipation

Urinary incontinence

Slight slowing of thought, memory, and thinking (however, delirium, dementia, and severe memory loss are NOT a normal part of aging)

Reduced reflexes and coordination and difficulty with balance

Decrease in visual acuity

Diminished peripheral vision

Some degree of hearing loss

Wrinkling and sagging skin

Whitening or graying of hair

Weight loss, after age 55 in men and after age 65 in women, in part due to loss of muscle tissue.

Following are examples of how aging affects some of our major body systems.

Cells, organs and tissues:

Cells become less able to divide

The telomeres—the ends of the chromosomes inside every cell—gradually get shorter until, finally, they get so short that the cell dies

Waste products accumulate

Connective tissue between the cells becomes stiffer

The maximum functional capacity of many organs decreases

Heart and blood vessels:

The wall of the heart gets thicker

Heart muscle become less efficient (working harder to pump the same amount of blood)

The aorta (the body's main artery) becomes thicker, stiffer, and less flexible

Many of the body's arteries, including arteries supplying blood to the heart and brain, slowly develop atherosclerosis, although the condition never becomes severe in some people

Vital signs:

It is harder for the body to control its temperature

Heart rate takes longer to return to normal after exercise

Bones, muscles, joints:

Bones become thinner and less strong

Joints become stiffer and less flexible

The cartilage and bone in joints starts to weaken

Muscle tissue becomes less bulky and less strong

Digestive system:

The movement of food through the digestive system becomes slower

The stomach, liver, pancreas, and small
intestine make smaller amounts of digestive
juices

Brain and nervous system:

The number of nerve cells in the brain and
spinal cord decreases.

The number of connections between nerve cells
decreases

Abnormal structures, known as plaques and
tangles, may form in the brain.

Eyes and Ears:

The retinas get thinner, the irises get stiffer

The lenses become less clear

The walls of the ear canal get thinner

The eardrums get thicker

Skin, nails, and hair:

Skin gets thinner and becomes less elastic

Sweat glands produce less sweat

Nails grow more slowly up

Chapter 3

why humans age.

How do we age? – The hallmarks of aging
There is much discussion among researchers about the mechanisms that contribute to the aging process. However, it is widely accepted that damage to genetic material, cells and tissues that accumulate with age and cannot be repaired by the body are causal factors for the functional decline associated with old age. But what causes this damage on the molecular level and why it can be repaired in young but not old organisms is much less clear.

To better characterize the aging process, scientists have started to identify and categorize the cellular and molecular hallmarks of aging. Nine candidate hallmarks are generally considered to contribute to the aging process and together determine the observable characteristics of aging. A corresponding process is considered a hallmark of aging, if its deterioration causes premature aging, while its

improvement ameliorates health during aging
and extends lifespan.

The nine hallmarks of aging:

1 Genomic instability
2 Telomere attrition
3 Epigenetic alterations
4 Loss of proteostasis
5 Deregulated nutrient sensing
6 Mitochondrial dysfunction
7 Cellular senescence
8 Stem cell exhaustion
9 Altered intercellular communication

The nine characteristics of aging clearly show
how complex the aging process is at the
molecular level and how it can be influenced in
many different ways. Although the knowledge
of aging research is constantly evolving, the
nine hallmarks of aging provide an excellent
basis for our knowledge of the fundamental
biology of aging.

Why do we age?

Evolutionary theories of aging
The nine hallmarks of aging provide a good
overview of the mechanisms that answer the
question of "how do we age?". But why do we
age at all? If there are processes in our cells that
can extend our lifespan, why have organisms
not developed mechanisms to do so?

Lifespan varies greatly between animals
ranging from only a few hours in mayflies up to
fivehundred years in Iceland clams. Some more
primitive animals like sea anemones and the
fresh-water polyp hydra do not seem to age at
all, while the longest-living vertebrate species is
the Greenland shark, that can live up to 400
years and only reaches sexual maturity at the
age of 150. However, aging is not the only
strategy developed during evolution, as some
animals like the giant pacific octopus, male ants
or males of the small marsupial Antechinus
agilis die immediately after reproduction. Thus,
although most organisms age the questions
"Why do we age?" and "What determines the

difference in longevity between species?" are much less understood.

From an evolutionary perspective aging is a paradox. aging makes us less healthy and why would such a deleterious process evolve? The answer is, aging evolves not because it is useful but as a side-effect of something else. This conclusion is derived from two popular aging theories proposed by evolutionary biologists Peter Medawar and George Williams already in the 1950s and 1960s.

The "mutation accumulation" theory by Peter Medawar states that the force of natural selection stays high until first reproduction. Afterwards, it declines with age. Therefore, deleterious mutations, whose effects only occur late in life, can accumulate because they are not selected against. This consideration is also termed the "selection shadow". This means that the most important goal of an organism is its reproduction and until that point natural selection ensures the maintenance of the cellular processes essential for survival. After reproduction, there is no evolutionary pressure to ensure the continued survival of the organism. Cellular processes decline, the organism ages and ultimately dies.The "antagonistic pleiotropy" theory by George Williams states that natural selection can favour gene variants with beneficial effects early in life, even if the same variants have detrimental effects later on. As the harmful effects of these genes only occur in old age after the reproductive phase, they have little evolutionary impact. Nature cannot directly select against a gene or its mutation that causes the death of an individual in old age, if its harmful effects do not occur before the end of the reproductive phase.

Another conclusion derived from these theories is that the intrinsic rate of aging of an organism is expected to evolve in accordance with the level of extrinsic hazard encountered. This means, the more likely an animal is to die due to predation or lack of food, the shorter-lived it usually is. Animals that developed strategies to avoid hazard are usually longer-lived. For example, birds and bats, which can escape hazardous situation by flying are often long-lived, other strategies include social organization, or protection via poison or armour.

In summary, aging only evolves as a side effect and therefore is not a programmed process like development, i.e. no genes evolved to cause damage and death. This may also explain why it is such a variable process within and between different individuals.

Chapter 4

Is there a cure for aging?

 Aging is not a disease to be cured of.

 Aging is the inevitable consequences of being alive.

The only way to prevent aging is by dying young. Aging should not be confused with the chronic disease we have come to associate with advanced age in Western society.

Therefore, we ought to be looking to eradicate chronic disease instead of trying to cure something that isn't an inllness.

Chapter 5

Causes of aging

Aging refers to the physiological changes we experience during our lifespan. It's also an inevitable part of life.

After all, our cells aren't made to last forever. The structures and functions in our cells decline over time.

HiBut why does this happen? For decades, scientists have been studying the subject. There are currently more than 300 theoriesTrusted Source on why we age, and experts are learning more every day.

Let's explore why humans age, and how you can slow down the effects.

Types of aging.

Aging can be categorized into two types and due to two types of factors, intrinsic and extrinsic.

Intrinsic aging vs. extrinsic aging

Intrinsic aging is a genetically predetermined process that occurs naturally.
Extrinsic aging is a result of outside factors chose by you, such as where you live, your stress levels, and your lifestyle habits (like smoking).

Cellular aging:
Cellular aging is due to intrinsic factors. It's related to the biological aging of cells.

Cells are the basic building blocks of the body. Your cells are programmed to divide, multiply, and perform basic biological functions.

But the more cells divide, the older they get. In turn, cells eventually lose their ability to function properly.

Cellular damage also increases as cells get older. This makes the cell less healthy, causing biological processes to fail. Cellular damage accumulates over time, too.

Damage-related and environmental aging
Damage-related and environmental aging is related to extrinsic factors. It refers to how our surroundings and lifestyle affect how we age.

This includes factors like:

air pollution
tobacco smoke
alcohol consumption
malnutrition
ultraviolet radiation (UV) exposure
Over time, these factors can damage our cells and contribute to aging.

Everyone experiences both types of aging. However, each form of aging varies from person to person, which explains why we age in different ways.

Theories on aging
It's generally accepted that aging is caused by multiple processes, rather than one reason. It's also likely that these processes interact and overlap with each other.

Here are some of the most prominent theories:

Programmed theories of aging.

Programmed aging theories say that people are designed to age and that our cells have a predetermined lifespan that's encoded into our bodies.

Also called active, or adaptive, aging theories, they include:

Gene theory.

This theory suggests that specific genes turn "on" and "off" over time, causing aging. Endocrine theory. According to this theory, aging is caused by changes in hormones, which are produced by the endocrine system. Immunological theory. Also called the autoimmune theory, this is the idea that the immune response is designed to decline. The result is disease and aging.
Programmed theories have many supporters. However, they suggest that habits linked to

longevity, like quitting smoking and exercise, are useless. This is likely inaccurate, as research has continuously proven that these habits affect life expectancy.

Error theories of aging.

Error theories, or damage theories, are the opposite of programmed theories. They hypothesize that aging is caused by cellular changes that are random and unplanned.

Error theories of aging include:

Wear and tear theory. This is the idea that cells break down and become damaged over time. But critics argue that it doesn't account for the body's ability to repair.

Genome instability theory. According to this theory, aging happens because the body loses its ability to repair DNA damage.

Cross-linkage theory. This theory claims that aging is due to the buildup of cross-linked proteins, which damages cells and slows biological functions.

Rate-of-living theory. Proponents of this theory say that an organism's rate of metabolism determines its lifespan. However, the theory lacks solid and consistent scientific evidence. Free radical theory. This theory suggests that aging is due to the buildup of oxidative stress, which is caused by free radicals. But some say this theory fails to explain other types of cellular damage seen in aging.

Mitochondrial theory. As a variation of the free radical theory, this theory says that mitochondrial damage releases free radicals and causes aging. The theory lacks hard scientific evidence.

Genetic theory of aging
The genetic theory proposes that aging primarily depends on genetics. In other words, our life expectancy is regulated by the genes we got from our parents.

Since genes have predetermined traits, it's thought this theory overlaps with programmed theories of aging.

Genetic theories include:

Telomere theory. Telomeres protect the ends of your chromosomes as they multiply. Over time, telomeres shorten, which is associated with disease and aging.

Programmed senescence theory. Cellular senescence occurs when cells stop dividing and growing, but don't die. This theory suggests that this causes aging.

Stem cell theory. Stem cells can turn into other cells, which helps repair tissue and organs. But the function of stem cells declines over time, potentially contributing to aging.

Longevity gene theory. This is the idea that certain genes extend lifespan. More research is necessary.

The limitation of genetic theories is that they disregard the importance of external factors. In fact, it's estimated that just 25 percentTrusted Source of lifespan is influenced by genetics. This suggests that environmental and lifestyle factors play a major role.

Evolutionary theory of aging
Natural selection refers to the adaptive traits of an organism. These traits can help the organism adjust to their environment, so they're more likely to survive.

According to evolutionary theories, aging is based on natural selection. It says that an organism begins aging after they have reached their peak of reproduction and have passed down adaptive traits.

Evolutionary theories include:

Mutation accumulation. This theory presumes that random mutations accumulate later in life.
Antagonistic pleiotropy. According to this theory, genes that promote fertility early in life have negative effects later on.
Disposable soma theory. The theory claims that when more metabolic resources are directed

toward reproduction, the less is put toward
DNA repair. The result is cell damage and
aging.
These theories are still being researched and
require more evidence.

Biochemical theory of aging
Another theory is that biochemical reactions
cause aging. These reactions occur naturally
and continuously throughout life.

This theory is rooted in various concepts,
including:

Advanced glycation end products (AGEs). AGEs
develop when fats or protein are exposed to
sugar. High levels may lead to oxidative stress,
which speeds up aging.
Heat shock response. Heat shock proteins
protect cells from stress, but their response
decreases as we age.
Damage accumulation. Normal chemical
reactions damage DNA, proteins, and
metabolites over time.

Chapter 6

Troubles of aging

Old age is a unique life phase characterized by various health, cognitive, emotional, social, and financial changes. Most people consider old age a problem-ridden stage of life, with aging problems usually occurring after 65.

Article Contents hide

1 Cognitive Problems
2 Emotional Problems
3 Social Problems
The four major old age problems include:

Physical problems
Cognitive problems
Emotional problems
Social problems

Physical problems

Physical decline and illness are one of the biggest problems aging people experience. Deteriorating health may prevent a person from doing things you enjoy or interfere with their routine activities. Also, chronic illness in the elderly may limit or cause a loss of independence, which is distressing for most people.

Cognitive Problems

Mental disorders and cognitive decline are often associated with old age. Aging adults are susceptible to dementia, psychotic depression, personality changes, mood swings, aggression, and other mental health issues.

Emotional Problems

The decline in health and mental ability makes aging people dependent. Lost independence can be a great source of stress. Additionally, many aging adults face emotional challenges such as feelings of loneliness and isolation. The death of a spouse and other loved ones can add to the

stress, depression, and anxiety the person
already experiences.

Social Problems

Transition to retirement often means limited
social life. Also, the death of a spouse, friends,
and relatives restricts the person's participation
in social life. Studies show that loneliness and
fear of being cut off from social circles are
among the biggest fears people have as they
age.

Chapter 7

15 healthy habits to a long life

Many people think that life expectancy is largely determined by genetics.

However, genes play a much smaller role than originally believed. It turns out that environmental factors like diet and lifestyle are key.

Here are 13 habits linked to a long life.

1. Avoid overeating.

The link between calorie intake and longevity currently generates a lot of interest.

Animal studies suggest that a 10–50% reduction in normal calorie intake may increase maximum lifespan.

Studies of human populations renowned for longevity also observe links between low calorie intake, an extended lifespan, and a lower likelihood of disease.

What's more, calorie restriction may help reduce excess body weight and belly fat, both of which are associated with shorter lifespans .

That said, long-term calorie restriction is often unsustainable and can include negative side effects, such as increased hunger, low body temperature, and a diminished sex drive.

Whether calorie restriction slows aging or extends your lifespan is not yet fully understood.

SUMMARY

Limitingyour calories may help you live longer and protect against disease. However, more human research is needed.

2. Eat more nuts.

Nuts are nutritional powerhouses.

They're rich in protein, fiber, antioxidants, and beneficial plant compounds. What's more, they're a great source of several vitamins and minerals, such as copper, magnesium, potassium, folate, niacin, and vitamins B6 and E.

Several studies show that nuts have beneficial effects on heart disease, high blood pressure, inflammation, diabetes, metabolic syndrome, belly fat levels, and even some forms of cancer.

One study found that people who consumed at least 3 servings of nuts per week had a 39% lower risk of premature death.

Similarly, two recent reviews including over 350,000 people noted that those who ate nuts had a 4–27% lower risk of dying during the study period — with the greatest reductions seen in those who ate 1 serving of nuts per day.

SUMMARY

Adding some nuts to your daily routine may keep you healthy and help you live longer.

3. Try out turmeric.

When it comes to anti-aging strategies, turmeric is a great option. That's because this spice contains a potent bioactive compound called curcumin.

Due to its antioxidant and anti-inflammatory properties, curcumin is thought to help maintain brain, heart, and lung function, as well as protect against cancers and age-related diseases.

Curcumin is linked to an increased lifespan in both insects and mice. However, these findings have not always been replicated, and no human studies are currently available.

Nevertheless, turmeric has been consumed for thousands of years in India and is generally considered safe.

SUMMARY

Curcumin, the main bioactive compound in
turmeric, has antioxidant and
anti-inflammatory properties. Some animal
studies
suggest that it can increase lifespan.

4. Eat plenty of healthy plant foods.

Consuming a wide variety of plant foods, such
as fruits, vegetables, nuts, seeds, whole grains,
and beans, may decrease disease risk and
promote longevity.

For example, many studies link a plant-rich diet
to a lower risk of premature death, as well as a
reduced risk of cancer, metabolic syndrome,
heart disease, depression, and brain
deterioration.
These effects are attributed to plant foods'
nutrients and antioxidants, which include
polyphenols, carotenoids, folate, and vitamin C.

Accordingly, several studies link vegetarian and
vegan diets, which are naturally higher in plant
foods, to a 12–15% lower risk of premature
death.

The same studies also report a 29–52% lower risk of dying from cancer or heart, kidney, or hormone-related diseases.

What's more, some research suggests that the risk of premature death and certain diseases increases with greater meat consumption.

However, other studies report either nonexistent or much weaker links — with the negative effects seeming specifically linked to processed meat.

Vegetarians and vegans also generally tend to be more health-conscious than meat eaters, which could at least partly explain these findings.

Overall, eating plenty of plant foods is likely to benefit health and longevity.

SUMMARY

Eating plenty of plant foods is likely to

help you live longer and lower your risk of various common diseases.

5. Stay physically active.

It should come as no surprise that staying physically active can keep you healthy and add years to your life.

As few as 15 minutes of exercise per day may help you achieve benefits, which could include an additional 3 years of life.

Furthermore, your risk of premature death may decrease by 4% for each additional 15 minutes of daily physical activity.

A recent review observed a 22% lower risk of early death in individuals who exercised — even though they worked out less than the recommended 150 minutes per week.

People who hit the 150-minute recommendation were 28% less likely to die early. What's more, that number was 35% for those who exercised beyond this guidance.

Finally, some research links vigorous activity to a 5% greater reduction in risk compared to low- or moderate-intensity activities.

SUMMARY

Regular physical activity can extend your lifespan. Exercising more than 150 minutes per week is best, but even small amounts can help.

6. Don't smoke.

Smoking is strongly linked to disease and early death..

Overall, people who smoke may lose up to 10 years of life and be 3 times more likely to die prematurely than those who never pick up a cigarettes.

Keep in mind that it's never too late to quit.

One study reports that individuals who quit smoking by age 35 may prolong their lives by up to 8.5 years.

Furthermore, quitting smoking in your 60s may add up to 3.7 years to your life. In fact, quitting in your 80s may still provide benefits.

SUMMARY

Stopping smoking can significantly prolong your life — and it's never too late to quit.

7. Moderate your alcohol intake.

Heavy alcohol consumption is linked to liver, heart, and pancreatic disease, as well as an overall increased risk of early death.

However, moderate consumption is associated with a reduced likelihood of several diseases, as well as a 17–18% decrease in your risk of premature death.

Wine is considered particularly beneficial due to its high content of polyphenol antioxidants.

Results from a 29-year study showed that men who preferred wine were 34% less likely to die early than those who preferred beer or spirits.

In addition, one review observed wine to be especially protective against heart disease, diabetes, neurological disorders, and metabolic syndrome.

To keep consumption moderate, it is recommended that women aim for 1–2 units or less per day and a maximum of 7 per week. Men should keep their daily intake to less than 3 units, with a maximum of 14 per week.

It's important to note that no strong research indicates that the benefits of moderate drinking are greater than those of abstaining from alcohol.

In other words, there is no need to start drinking if you don't usually consume alcohol.

SUMMARY

If you drink alcohol, maintaining a moderate intake may help prevent disease and prolong your life. Wine may be particularly beneficial.

8. Prioritize your happiness.

Feeling happy can significantly increase your longevity.

In fact, happier individuals had a 3.7% reduction in early death over a 5-year study period.

A study of 180 Catholic nuns analyzed their self-reported levels of happiness when they first entered the monastery and later compared these levels to their longevity.

Those who felt happiest at 22 years of age were 2.5 times more likely to still be alive six decades later.

Finally, a review of 35 studies showed that happy people may live up to 18% longer than their less happy counterparts.

SUMMARY

 Happiness likely has positive effects not only for your mood but also your lifespan.

9. Avoid chronic stress and anxiety.

Anxiety and stress may significantly decrease your lifespan.

For instance, women suffering from stress or anxiety are reportedly up to two times more likely to die from heart disease, stroke, or lung cancer.

Similarly, the risk of premature death is up to three times higher for anxious or stressed men compared to their more relaxed counterparts (If you're feeling stressed, laughter and optimism could be two key components of the solution.

Studies show that pessimistic individuals have a 42% higher risk of early death than more optimistic people. However, both laughter and

a positive outlook on life can reduce stress,
potentially prolonging your life.

SUMMARY

Finding ways to reduce your anxiety and stress
levels can extend your lifespan.
Maintaining an optimistic outlook on life can be
beneficial, too.

10. Nurture your social circle.

Researchers report that maintaining healthy
social networks can help you live up to 50%
longer.

In fact, having just 3 social ties may decrease
your risk of early death by more than 200%.

Studies also link healthy social networks to
positive changes in heart, brain, hormonal, and
immune function, which may decrease your risk
of chronic diseases.

A strong social circle might also help you react less negatively to stress, perhaps further explaining the positive effect on lifespan.

Finally, one study reports that providing support to others may be more beneficial than receiving it. In addition to accepting care from your friends and family, make sure to return the favor.

SUMMARY

 Nurturing close relationships may result in decreased stress levels, improved immunity, and an extended lifespan.

11. Be more conscientious.

Conscientiousness refers to a person's ability to be self-disciplined, organized, efficient, and goal-oriented.

Based on data from a study that followed 1,500 boys and girls into old age, kids who were considered persistent, organized, and

disciplined lived 11% longer than their less
conscientious counterparts.

Conscientious people may also have lower
blood pressure and fewer psychiatric
conditions, as well as a lower risk of diabetes
and heart or joint problems.

This might be partly because conscientious
individuals are less likely to take dangerous
risks or react negatively to stress — and more
likely to lead successful professional lives or be
responsible about their health.

Conscientiousness can be developed at any
stage in life through steps as small as tidying up
a desk, sticking to a work plan, or being on
time.

SUMMARY

Being conscientious is associated with a longer
lifespan and fewer health problems in
old age.

12. Drink coffee or tea.

Both coffee and tea are linked to a decreased risk of chronic disease.

For instance, the polyphenols and catechins found in green tea may decrease your risk of cancer, diabetes, and heart disease.

Similarly, coffee is linked to a lower risk of type 2 diabetes, heart disease, and certain cancers and brain ailments, such as Alzheimer's and Parkinson's.

Additionally, both coffee and tea drinkers benefit from a 20–30% lower risk of early death compared to non-drinkers.

Just remember that too much caffeine can also lead to anxiety and insomnia, so you may want to curb your intake to the recommended limit of 400 mg per day — around 4 cups of coffee.

It's also worth noting that it generally takes six hours for caffeine's effects to subside. Therefore, if you have trouble getting enough high-quality sleep, you may want to shift your intake to earlier in the day.

SUMMARY

Moderate consumption of tea and coffee may benefit healthy aging and longevity.

13. Develop a good sleeping pattern.

Sleep is crucial for regulating cell function and helping your body heal.

A recent study reports that longevity is likely linked to regular sleeping patterns, such as going to bed and waking up around the same time each day.

Sleep duration also seems to be a factor, with both too little and too much being harmful.

For instance, sleeping less than 5–7 hours per night is linked to a 12% greater risk of early death, while sleeping more than 8–9 hours per night could also decrease your lifespan by up to 38%.

Too little sleep may also promote inflammation and increase your risk of diabetes, heart disease, and obesity. These are all linked to a shortened lifespan.

On the other hand, excessive sleep could be linked to depression, low physical activity, and undiagnosed health conditions, all of which may negatively affect your lifespan.

SUMMARY

Developing a sleep routine that includes 7–8 hours of sleep each night may help you live longer.

14. Forgive

Letting go of grudges has surprising physical health benefits. Chronic anger is linked to heart disease, stroke, poorer lung health, and other problems. Forgiveness will reduce anxiety, lower blood pressure, and help you breathe more easily. The rewards tend to go up as you get older.

15. Get spiritual.

People who attend religious services tend to live longer than those who don't. In a 12-year study of people over age 65, those who went more than once a week had higher levels of a key immune system protein than their peers who didn't. The strong social network that develops among people who worship together may boost your health.

The bottom line

Longevity may seem beyond your control, but
many healthy habits may lead you to a ripe, old
age.

These include drinking coffee or tea, exercising,
getting enough sleep, and limiting your alcohol
intake.

Taken together, these habits can boost your
health and put you on the path to a long life.

Conflicting information out there, there is not
much of a one-size-fits-all plan, and there's also
a very wide range of quality standards within
dietary supplements," she added.

That's why she encourages people to work with
a dietitian to learn if they have any nutrient
deficiencies, and make an individualized plan to
meet their particular needs.